The Every Day Keto Diet Book

Quick and Delicious Recipes For a Healthy Lifestyle incl. Breakfast, Meal Prep, Dinner & Snacks

Marc C. Goodwin

ISBN - 9798799742485

Table of Contents

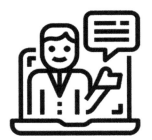

Introduction

If you want to try the keto diet and you aren't sure where to start, you'll be pleased to learn that there are a plethora of different recipes that you can whip up very quickly and easily, without slaving in the kitchen for hours after a busy day at work. This book is going to run through some super simple options, as well as a few more luxurious ones so you can treat yourself when you have a bit more time and energy for cooking.

What Is The Ketogenic Diet?

The ketogenic diet (keto for short) has become extremely popular in recent years, and it is a strict, low-carb diet that aims to put the body into a state of ketosis. The term covers several other diets, including low carb, high fat diets, the Dukan diet, and the Atkins diet.

If you aren't sure what the body being put into a state of ketosis actually means, let's start by exploring that. Normally, your body uses the carbohydrates in your food to create energy. It converts the glucose in these carbohydrates, and burns the glucose to make the energy to fuel our muscles and basic functions.

However, if the body does not have access to enough glucose, it looks for energy elsewhere. This means that the liver will start to break down the stores of fat in the body, and use these to make energy instead – and this is what happens if you don't eat any carbohydrates for a while. The body has to start tapping into your fat reserves and using them up instead. This diet is therefore popular for cutting down on excess fat and reducing your weight.

What Are The Advantages Of Following A Keto Diet?

The keto diet started as a medical diet, and it is still used to treat certain conditions like epilepsy, but this must be done with great care because it can be dangerous. On the whole, the main advantage associated with the ketogenic diet and ketosis is weight loss, and this is why most people decide to give this diet a go.

Some people find that they feel more energised and healthier on this diet, and many find that their overall appetite is reduced, which can help to sustain weight loss in the future. A well managed ketogenic diet may also help followers to reduce their blood sugar, their blood pressure, and their cholesterol, so many people can benefit from this sort of eating in a whole multitude of different ways.

What Are The Top Tips For Succeeding On A Keto Diet?

The most important thing to know about the keto diet is that it's about avoiding carbs as much as possible, so to follow it, you will need to count the number of carbohydrates that you are consuming in a day, and keep the number as low as you can. Often, you will be aiming to consume less than 50 grams of carbohydrates per day, although this will depend upon your situation and general health.

Of course, counting your carbs constantly is often a frustrating process and it's challenging to keep it up in the long term – but this shouldn't be too much of an issue. With time, you will get a good idea of which foods are and are not suitable for this sort of diet, and you'll be able to make estimates in your head without needing to think about the numbers in too much detail. In the early stages, however, you will need to be tracking the numbers if you want to be successful.

Another top tip for success is to start exercising frequently. Because this means that your body will burn more energy, it will help you get into a state of ketosis more quickly, and will burn off fat much faster. You should be aware, however, that it takes time for your body to adjust to the new method of fuelling itself, and you may find that your performance is reduced for the first few weeks. Do not push too hard, or you could injure yourself.

What Can't You Eat On A Ketogenic Diet?

Only certain foods are allowed if you are following a ketogenic diet. You won't be surprised to hear that most carbohydrate-rich foods are out. These include rice, baked goods, bread, and pasta, but the diet also means cutting back on or avoiding starchy vegetables like potatoes, certain fruits, and legumes.

If you have just started on this diet, you might find that a pretty limiting restriction, and it can make it very difficult to find foods that are appealing, balanced, and healthy. If you're struggling in the kitchen, this book is here to help. It's crucial to make sure that you are replacing carbohydrates with other forms of energy, or you may make yourself ill through deficiencies.

What Can You Eat On A Ketogenic Diet?

Nuts, some fruits such as berries, and leafy greens are popular options for the keto diet. However, a lot of fruits and vegetables are high in carbohydrates, and most of your diet will depend heavily on eating fats. Often, you will find that your diet becomes heavy in meat and fish, as well as eggs and dairy.

You may also eat a lot of peppers, squashes, and high-fat foods like avocados and olives.

We'll cover the foods in a lot more detail throughout the recipes below, but that should give you some idea of what a keto dish might look like. Remember, carbohydrates must be low, so many fruits are out — a single banana can contain around 27 grams of carbohydrates, and most people on this diet are aiming to be below 50 grams at the most.

How Quickly Will I Achieve Ketosis?

It usually takes a few days to reach ketosis, because your body will still be burning up energy from carbohydrates for a while. Be patient, and be prepared to feel a little odd for a few days when you first begin a keto diet; some major changes will be occurring in how your body processes food.

Are There Any Medical Risks Associated With This Diet?

It is thought that ketosis is a process that humans evolved to help themselves survive famines. In today's world, most keto diets involve eating moderately high protein, high fat foods, and you should always consult with your doctor before starting a new diet — especially one as restrictive as the ketogenic diet. People with certain health conditions could suffer from undesired results and may even make themselves ill, so always talk to a medical professional before starting a new diet to minimise your risk of issues.

It is important to keep your liver health up while following this diet, so try to focus on foods that help this organ out – onions and garlic are good choices. You should also cut back on things like alcohol, sugar, and caffeine. If you suffer from any liver problems, take particular care to consult with your doctor. Diabetics and people with kidney disease should be similarly cautious.

You should also be aware that ketosis can cause certain symptoms when you first embark upon this diet, and you may need to push through these in order to continue with it. Headaches, fatigue, a dry mouth, and nausea are all common issues, but most of these can be overcome by ensuring that you drink enough water and balance your diet with care.

It is also a good idea to include plenty of foods that are good for your guts to help keep your digestive system operating properly – because a keto diet often lacks fibre. Choose live yogurt, leafy greens, and fermented vegetables to supplement your meals.

If you find that you suffer negative side effects from following a ketogenic diet and these do not quickly resolve themselves, or they seem to get worse as you continue with the diet, it is important to cease and talk to a medical professional about your experience. This book is not intended to offer medical advice; it will simply supply recipes that you may find help you on your weight loss journey.

Healthy Keto Breakfast Recipes

For many people, breakfast is the most important meal of the day, and it's also one that a lot of people struggle with. When you've just dragged yourself out of bed with a long day looming ahead of you, you may not feel like hitting the kitchen – but it's important to give your body some fuel to run on, or you'll be setting yourself up for failure.

In this section, we're going to cover some simple breakfast recipes, and a few more decadent recipes for the days when you feel like spoiling yourself. Remember, keto food doesn't need to be boring or tasteless, and these breakfasts should wow you!

Avocado And Strawberry Smoothie

If you struggle to get a proper meal down first thing, this is a perfect alternative – breakfast in a cup. This recipe only has three ingredients, and it's very easy to adjust the quantities to better suit your tastes. This should make enough for five servings, so feel free to make more or less, depending on your preferences.

Serves: 5

You will need:

♦ 1 large avocado

♦ 450 g / 1 lb. of frozen (or fresh) strawberries

♦ 370 ml / 1.5 cups of unsweetened almond milk

Method:

1. Slice the avocado in half and remove the stone, and then scoop the flesh from the skins and discard them.

2. If you are using fresh strawberries, rinse the fruits and remove the tops.

3. Add all of the ingredients to the blender and blend for 4 minutes, or until smooth.

4. Place in the fridge until chilled, and then consume.

Approximate Nutritional Information For One Serving:

Calories: 125

Fat: 8.9 g

Saturated Fat: 1.7 g

Cholesterol: 0 mg

Sodium: 59 mg

Total Carbohydrates: 11.8 g

Dietary Fibre: 4.8 g

Total Sugars: 5.5 g

Protein: 1.1 g

Tofu Twist On Scrambled Eggs

For those who don't enjoy eggs in the morning, keto breakfasts can be challenging, but you can still have a variation on the classic scrambled eggs by swapping it for tofu. If you like the sound of this, you'll love tofu scrambled eggs, and the great news is that these are almost as quick and easy as real scrambled eggs. Skip the bread to ensure that this recipe is keto, and just enjoy your scrambled "eggs" tofu as it comes.

Serves: 2

You will need:

- 1 tablespoon of olive oil

- 1/2 teaspoon of turmeric

- 1 teaspoon of smoked paprika

- 1/2 teaspoon of cumin

- 2 cloves of garlic

- 1 onion

- 100 g / 3.5 oz of cherry tomatoes

- 250 g / 8.8 oz of firm tofu
- Herbs of your choice (optional)

Method:

1. Begin by slicing your onion into thin rings, and crushing or mincing the garlic cloves. Next, halve your cherry tomatoes.

2. Warm the oil in a pan over a medium heat, and then add the onion and fry for about eight minutes until it turns golden. Add the spices and the garlic, and cook for a minute or two, until fragrant. Do not let the garlic burn.

3. In a separate bowl, mash the tofu into chunks, with some finer pieces.

4. Tip the tofu mash into the pan and fry gently for a few minutes.

5. Add the tomato halves and stir, frying gently for around five minutes, until the tomatoes have started to soften and turn golden.

6. Stir in any herbs that you wish to include, and serve steaming hot.

Approximate Nutritional Information For One Serving:

Calories: 190

Fat: 12.7 g

Saturated Fat: 2.1 g

Cholesterol: 0 mg

Sodium: 22 mg

Total Carbohydrates: 11.4 g

Dietary Fibre: 3.5 g

Total Sugars: 4.6 g

Protein: 11.8g

Porridge / Oatmeal Turned Keto

You unfortunately can't eat oats on the ketogenic diet, and this leaves a lot of people lost on what to have for breakfast, because porridge / oatmeal is such a classic and simple option. If your go-to start to the day is porridge / oatmeal, you will need to get a little inventive to continue enjoying it, but fortunately, it is still possible! You'll use a fair chunk of your daily carbs on this recipe, but if you're someone who needs a filling breakfast for the start of the day, it's perfect.

Serves: 1

You will need:

- ◆ 2 tablespoons of double cream (heavy cream)
- ◆ 2 tablespoons of flaxseed
- ◆ 1 tablespoon of coconut flour
- ◆ ½ teaspoon of vanilla essence (or a little more for more flavour)
- ◆ 115 ml / ½ cup of unsweetened almond milk

Method:

1. Place a saucepan on the stove and turn the heat to medium.
2. Add your flaxseed and coconut flour to the pan, and then mix in the double cream, the vanilla essence, and the almond milk.
3. Stir the ingredients together and heat gently for about 10 to 15 minutes, stirring to prevent the mixture from sticking to the bottom of the pan. It should become thick and creamy.
4. When it is hot in the centre, serve and enjoy immediately. You can add sugar-free maple syrup, chopped nuts, or berries if you want to increase the interest of this meal, or eat it plain.

Approximate Nutritional Information For One Serving:

Calories: 300
Fat: 20.9 g
Saturated Fat: 9 g
Cholesterol: 41 mg
Sodium: 105 mg
Total Carbohydrates: 18.1 g
Dietary Fibre: 12.2 g
Total Sugars: 0.6 g
Protein: 7 g

Omelette

Eggs are a great option for keto diets, because they are high in protein and very filling, and most people find they make an excellent breakfast. The great news is that you can enjoy eggs and plenty of other fillings with an omelette, and you won't even miss the bread. They're also super quick, which is ideal if you're heading out to work or having a lazy Saturday together.

Serves: 1

You will need:

- ♦ 2 large eggs
- ♦ 30 g / 1 oz. of bacon
- ♦ 60 g / 2 oz. of deli turkey
- ♦ 2 tablespoons of cream cheese
- ♦ 2 teaspoons of tinned chopped tomatoes
- ♦ ½ teaspoon of butter (unsalted)

Method:

1. Start by cooking your bacon, and then chop the meat (both bacon and turkey) into small cubes once it is ready.

2. Melt your butter gently in a large skillet over a low or medium heat, being careful not to burn it. Whip up the eggs until they are frothy, and then add them to the skillet once the butter is hot.

3. Allow the eggs to cook for a few moments, and then tip the tomatoes, the cream cheese, the turkey, and the bacon onto one side of the omelette, but not the other (this will allow you to fold it over later).

4. Allow it a few more moments to cook, and slip your spatula under the side of the omelette without the filling. Flip it over on top of the filling, and leave it for a few minutes while it cooks and warms the ingredients. The cream cheese should start to melt.

5. Flip the omelette so that the other side is face down against the pan and give it another minute or two of cooking, and then serve piping hot. If you like, add a sprinkle of dried basil or parsley for some extra flavour.

Approximate Nutritional Information For One Serving:

Calories: 461

Fat: 33.2 g

Saturated Fat: 12.9 g

Cholesterol: 465 mg

Sodium: 1626 mg

Total Carbohydrates: 6.6 g

Dietary Fibre: 0.3 g

Total Sugars: 3.4 g

Protein: 33.4 g

Baked Eggs With Tomato

For those who enjoy eggs but don't fancy an omelette or would like a change from the standard options, these baked eggs are a gorgeous alternative. The best part is that you can add any herbs or spices you fancy to keep the flavour interesting and ensure your breakfast is satisfying. These eggs are filling, but the tomato lends them a fresher edge than many of the greasy breakfast options. It's a good idea to use really high quality tomatoes to maximise the flavour of this dish.

Serves: 4

You will need:

♦ 4 cloves of garlic

♦ 3 tablespoons of olive oil

♦ 2 tablespoons of chives or an alternative herb of your choice (try sage, parsley, oregano, thyme, or a mix)

♦ 900 g / 1.9 lb of fresh, ripe tomatoes (use small ones for sweetness)

♦ 4 eggs

Method:

1. Wash your tomatoes and cut them into halves or thick slices (halves will do for small tomatoes such as cherry tomatoes, but if you are using bigger tomatoes, cut them into chunks around a quarter of an inch thick).

2. Preheat your oven to 200 degrees C / 390 degrees F.

3. Spread the tomatoes in an oven-safe dish.

4. Peel and mince your garlic, and stir it into the tomatoes.

5. Drizzle the olive oil across the mixture, and then stir until everything is combined.

6. Bake in the oven for 40 minutes, until your tomatoes are lightly golden and very soft. Use a wooden spatula to make four hollows among the tomatoes, and break an egg into each one.

7. Cover the dish with foil and return it to the oven for another 7 minutes. Check that you are happy with the eggs' consistency, and then remove from the oven.

8. Add the chopped chives and serve hot.

Approximate Nutritional Information For One Serving:

Calories: 198

Fat: 15.4 g

Saturated Fat: 2.9 g

Cholesterol: 164 mg

Sodium: 73 mg

Total Carbohydrates: 10.2 g

Dietary Fibre: 2.8 g

Total Sugars: 6.3 g

Protein: 7.8 g

Keto Crepes

You might feel more like a luxury breakfast sometimes, and if so, there's a great option for you – keto crepes. Normal crepes are not suitable for the keto diet, but fortunately, it's easy to make ultra light and fluffy crepes that fit in perfectly by using almond flour instead. Just follow the directions below and choose some keto friendly toppings, such as a suitable sweetener, mashed avocado, cheese, or cooked meat.

Serves: 8

You will need:

♦ 70 g / ³/4 of a cup of fine almond flour (not almond meal, or your pancakes will come out gritty)

♦ 4 large eggs

♦ 115 g / 4 oz. of softened cream cheese

♦ 1 ¹/2 tablespoons of SPLENDA Sugar Blend for Baking

♦ 60 ml / ¹/4 of a cup of almond milk (unsweetened)

♦ Enough oil or butter to grease the pan in between crepes

Method:

1. Add your almond flour, sweetener, eggs, cream cheese, and almond milk to a blender, with a pinch of salt if you desire. Blend them until the whole mixture is smooth and completely combined.

2. Allow the mixture to rest for at least 5 minutes, and in the meantime, warm a large skillet over a medium heat. Lightly grease the skillet with just enough butter to cover the bottom, and then scoop 3 or 4 tablespoons of batter (or more for larger crepes) into the pan and tip the skillet to spread the crepe out. You want the crepes to be ultra thin and light, as this will ensure that they cook properly and come out soft.

3. Cook for a few minutes, and once the edges are starting to come loose from the pan, use a spatula to gently free the crepe. Slip the spatula beneath the crepe, being careful not to tear it, and then flip it onto the other side. You can also toss it in the pan if you are confident doing this, but be careful it doesn't end up on the floor!

4. Cook the other side until it is lightly brown, and then serve the crepe. Top it with whatever you choose, as long as it is keto-friendly. You might fancy a few berries, a little sugar-free chocolate spread, or some chopped bacon bits – the choice is yours!

5. If you want to make lots of crepes at once, place them on a baking tray in a warm oven to keep the temperature up. Crepes can be reheated, but they are nicest when cooked and eaten fresh.

Approximate Nutritional Information For One Crepe:

Calories: 116 g

Fat: 8.9 g

Saturated Fat: 4 g

Cholesterol: 109 mg

Sodium: 84 mg

Total Carbohydrates: 4.2 g

Dietary Fibre: 0.3 g

Total Sugars: 3.3 g

Protein: 4.8 g

Mushroom, Spinach, and Cheddar Cheese Casserole

If you're vegetarian, you might find it even harder to come up with good breakfast recipes, as a lot of these depend upon meat to make you feel full. Obviously, you can go for smoothies or chia pudding, but it's nice to have a hearty option up your sleeve for cold winter days and particularly hungry mornings.

The great thing about this casserole is it makes multiple servings, so you can share with friends or family, or you can put it in the fridge for the next day – win win on all sides. It's also easy to adjust the recipe to include other ingredients if you prefer, so long as you remember to account for any carbs that you add.

Serves: 12

You will need:

- ◆ 17 large eggs

- ◆ 2 onions

- ◆ 4 cloves of garlic

- ◆ 1 tablespoon of olive oil

- ◆ 450 g / 16 ounces of mushrooms

- ◆ 120 g / 4 cups of spinach leaves

- ◆ 115 g / 4 oz. of cheddar cheese (or other cheese if you prefer)

- ◆ 120 ml / ½ cup of whole milk

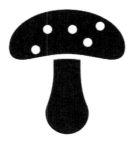

Method:

1. Start by thoroughly washing your spinach leaves and setting them aside to dry. Next, slice the mushrooms and the onions into thin strips, and mince your garlic.

2. Grate the cheddar cheese and measure out your other ingredients.

3. Grease a large baking tray with butter and preheat your oven to 175 degrees C / 350 degrees F.

4. Heat the olive oil in a large skillet over a high heat and add the mushrooms. Cook until lightly browned, and then stir in the garlic and the spinach. Cook until the spinach has wilted.

5. Tip the vegetable mix into the prepared baking dish and spread it out, and then spread the sliced onions across the top.

6. Sprinkle half of the cheddar cheese on top of the vegetables.

7. In a separate bowl, whisk your milk and eggs together, and season with salt and pepper if you wish to.

8. Pour the egg mix over the vegetables and cheese, and then sprinkle the other half of the cheddar cheese on top of this.

9. Transfer to the oven and bake for 40 minutes, checking at the 30 minute mark. The eggs should turn golden and pull away from the edges of the baking tray slightly.

10. Remove from the oven and use a knife blade inserted in the centre to check that the eggs have cooked through. They should not be remotely wobbly. Allow to cool for a few minutes, and then cut into squares and serve hot. It is also nice when eaten cold, so put some in the fridge for future breakfasts.

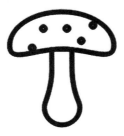

Approximate Nutritional Information For One Serving:

Calories: 163

Fat: 11.1 g

Saturated Fat: 4.3 g

Cholesterol: 243 mg

Sodium: 162 mg

Total Carbohydrates: 4.7 g

Dietary Fibre: 1 g

Total Sugars: 2.5 g

Protein: 12.3 g

Healthy Lunch Recipes

Lunch can be a tricky meal to manage too, because it often has quite specific requirements. You might need a lunch that is portable, a lunch that is easy to reheat, a lunch that can be eaten cold, or a lunch that is super quick to make – and possible all of these. We're going to cover some top recipes to make sure you're getting enough fuel in the middle of the day, so you don't end up running on an empty tank.

Lunch can be a particularly tricky meal because many of the go-to options that people depend on either use bread, wraps, potatoes, or pasta. Sandwiches, burritos, potato salad, and pasta salad are all out when it comes to following a keto diet, and if you're feeling totally stuck on what to eat instead, it's no surprise.

Let's get started on some great lunch recipes for you to try.

Coconut And Shrimp Soup

Soup is one of the best meals you can choose, and this Thai-like soup is delicious, filling, healthy – and low on carbs, making it perfect for a keto diet. One of the best things about soup is that you can make it in big batches, refrigerate it or freeze it, and easily reheat it any time you need.

Even if you have to take lunch to work, as long as you have access to a microwave, you can enjoy some piping hot soup and know that you're eating a healthy, balanced meal.

Serves: 2

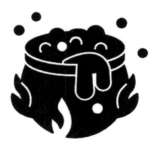

You will need:

- ◆ 400 ml / 1.7 cups of coconut milk

- ◆ 250 g / 8.8 oz of courgette / zucchini

- ◆ 150 g / 5.3 oz of cooked shrimps

- ◆ 3 tablespoons of Thai green curry paste

- ◆ 1 tablespoon of low-flavour oil (e.g. vegetable oil)

Method:

1. Shred the courgette / zucchini using a spiraliser to get long, thin strands.

2. Warm the oil over a medium heat and then cook the curry paste into it.

3. Add the coconut milk to the pan, and bring it to a low boil. Allow it to cook for a couple of minutes.

4. Add the shrimps and the spiralised courgette strands, and cook for another two minutes.

5. Check that the courgette is tender, and then serve piping hot.

Approximate Nutritional Information For One Serving:

Calories: 405

Fat: 34.9 g

Saturated Fat: 29 g

Cholesterol: 105 mg

Sodium: 377 mg

Total Carbohydrates: 12.3 g

Dietary Fibre: 4.6 g

Total Sugars: 6.3 g

Protein: 15.7 g

Baked Salmon With Lemon And Cream Cheese

For lunches at home, baked salmon is a wonderful keto option that manages to be both healthy and decadent. This recipe is super succulent and can be made with very little effort. You can choose any vegetables that you like as an accompaniment, but stay away from the carbohydrate-rich ones like carrots and potatoes.

Serves: 4

You will need:

- ◆ 1 tablespoon of butter
- ◆ 4 salmon fillets
- ◆ 4 slices of lemon
- ◆ 40 g / 1.4 oz. cream cheese to serve
- ◆ Broccoli, green beans, or another keto-friendly vegetable (optional, not included in nutritional information)

Method:

1. Melt the tablespoon of butter in the microwave or on the stove.

2. Remove the skins from the salmon fillets.

3. Place the salmon fillets in an oven-proof dish and brush with the melted butter.

4. Put the dish in the oven at 180 degrees C / 350 degrees F and bake for about 10 minutes.

5. Open the oven and place a slice of lemon on each fillet and then bake for another 10 minutes, or until tender (larger fillets will take longer). The salmon should be cooked through and flaky, with the lemon lightly brown on top. Remove the lemon if it starts to burn before the fish has finished cooking.

6. About 10 minutes before the fish is due to come out of the oven, steam the vegetables, and then serve everything with a square of cream cheese.

Approximate Nutritional Information For One Serving:

Calories: 343

Fat: 18.9 g

Saturated Fat: 6 g

Cholesterol: 128 mg

Sodium: 136 mg

Total Carbohydrates: 0.9 g

Dietary Fibre: 0.2 g

Total Sugars: 0.2 g

Protein: 40.1 g

Buffalo Shrimp Wraps Done In Lettuce

For those who find that they are missing out on a more filling "wrapped" lunch, using large leaves of lettuce is a great alternative. Since many sandwiches would contain lettuce anyway, using it to bundle up your favourite fillings is one way to continue enjoying your best lunches without the issue of bread. If you're stuck on what to fill the "wrap" with, why not try some buffalo shrimp?

Serves: 4

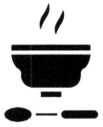

You will need:

- 1 tablespoon of olive oil

- 4 cloves of garlic

- ¼ of a tablespoon of butter

- 120 ml / ½ cup of hot sauce (or less if you prefer less heat; this will create quite a spicy dish)

- 1 head of Romaine lettuce

- 1 stick of celery

- 1 red onion

- 450 g / 1 lb. of shrimp

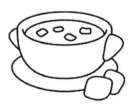

Method:

1.   Mince the garlic and chop the onion and celery into small, thin pieces.

2.   Peel, devein, and remove the tails of your shrimps.

3.   Add the butter to a saucepan and lightly fry the garlic for around a minute, and then add the hot sauce to the pan and stir the two together. Turn the heat down or off while you finish preparing the other ingredients.

4.   Add the olive oil to a large pan and warm it gently, and then add the shrimp. Cook for a couple of minutes on one side, and then flip them and cook for another 2 minutes. Once the shrimps are all opaque, turn the heat off and pour the buffalo sauce on top of them. Toss the shrimps until they are thoroughly coated.

5.   Wash your lettuce leaves and place them on a plate, and then add a scoop of shrimp and sauce, and then sprinkle some onion and celery on top. You can also include a little cheese with the meal if you want to.

Approximate Nutritional Information For One Serving:

Calories: 201

Fat: 6.5 g

Saturated Fat: 1.6 g

Cholesterol: 239 mg

Sodium: 1066 mg

Total Carbohydrates: 8.5 g

Dietary Fibre: 1.4 g

Total Sugars: 2.5 g

Protein: 26.7 g

Sausage And Egg Muffins

Sometimes, you need a lunch that's quick and easy to transport, and one that you can eat cold or heat up if you have the opportunity – and it needs to taste great either way. That is a lot to ask from a meal, especially when you add keto into the mix, but it can be done. You can use these fantastic muffins as a breakfast option, or toss one in your work lunch box and have it hot or cold, depending on how the day pans out.

It's a good idea to make these the night before and then store them in your fridge if you want to have them for lunch, unless you have a lot of free time in the mornings. Although they are a pretty simple recipe, they do take about 40 minutes to make because you have to account for the baking time.

Serves: 12

You will need:

- ♦ 115 g / 4 oz. of cream cheese

- ♦ 3 eggs

- ♦ 3 cloves of garlic

- ♦ 120 g / 1 cup of grated cheddar cheese

- ♦ ½ teaspoon of baking powder

- ♦ 30 g / 1/3 of a cup of almond flour

- ♦ 450 g / 1 lb. of breakfast sausage

Method:

1. Grate your cheddar cheese and mince the garlic.

2. Preheat your oven to 180 degrees C / 350 degrees F.

3. Put a skillet over a medium heat and add the breakfast sausage to it. Use a spatula to break the meat up, and then stir it in the pan until cooked. Set it aside once it is ready.

4. Add the cream cheese to a large mixing bowl and then mix in the sausage once it has cooled down. Stir thoroughly until totally combined, and then check that the mix is lukewarm or cool before moving on to the next step.

5. Beat the eggs and then add them to the sausage and cream cheese mixture. Stir in the cheese, the almond flour, the garlic, and finally the baking powder, and make sure everything is well mixed.

6. Place in the fridge and leave to chill for about 10 minutes. In the meantime, grease a muffin tray.

7. When the mix has chilled, use a teaspoon or other scoop to add small balls of the mixture to each of the muffin holes, and then transfer to the oven and bake for up to 20 minutes. The outside should become golden and the mixture should puff up.

8. Either serve hot, or cool the muffins and transfer them to an airtight container in the fridge. To reheat, microwave in 20 second bursts, or enjoy them cold. These muffins should also freeze well.

Approximate Nutritional Information For One Serving:

Calories: 228

Fat: 19.2

Saturated Fat: 8 g

Cholesterol: 93 mg

Sodium: 388 mg

Total Carbohydrates: 1.2 g

Dietary Fibre: 0.2 g

Total Sugars: 0.2 g

Protein: 12.3

Parmesan And Cauliflower Rice

Rice is a firm no on the keto diet, so it's well worth trying out cauliflower rice, which is a delicious and low carb alternative. You will need to mince the cauliflower pretty finely for this recipe, but the good news is that it cooks quickly and will give you a delicious, filling meal that is totally free from grains and low on carbs.

You can use this in pretty much any dish that would usually require rice, or you can just eat it as a meal in itself – it's a very flexible option. You can also make broccoli rice if you prefer that to cauliflower.

Serves: 4

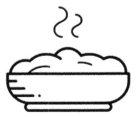

You will need:

- ♦ 2 tablespoons of double (heavy) cream

- ♦ 1 tablespoon of olive oil

- ♦ 1 tablespoon of butter

- ♦ 80 g / 2/3 of a cup of red pepper

- ♦ 2 onions

- ♦ ½ a cauliflower

- ♦ 1 stock cube

- ♦ 30 g / ¼ of a cup of Parmesan (or vegetarian Italian hard cheese)

Method:

1. If you have a food processor, add your cauliflower and turn it to "shred" mode to mince it into small pieces. You can do this by hand, but it will be slower and you will probably end up with larger chunks.

2. Add the cauliflower to a pan and add about 1 cm of water to the bottom. Add a stock cube, then place the pan on a medium heat and simmer it until the cauliflower turns tender.

3. Finely slice the onion and red pepper, and then add the butter and oil to a skillet and lightly fry the vegetables over a medium heat until they turn soft.

4. Either drain the cauliflower rice or leave the juice in. Add the Parmesan, double cream, and other vegetables and cook lightly for a few minutes, stirring well. Serve steaming hot, and consider adding a poached egg to the finished meal for a bit of velvety richness.

Approximate Nutritional Information For One Serving:

Calories: 157

Fat: 11 g

Saturated Fat: 5.1 g

Cholesterol: 23 mg

Sodium: 117 mg

Total Carbohydrates: 11.8 g

Dietary Fibre: 3.3 g

Total Sugars: 5.3 g

Protein: 5.1 g

Healthy Keto Dinner Recipes

To many people, dinner is the most important meal of the day, and it's the one that we often put the most time and energy into preparing. However, it can also be a challenge, because it is usually the time when the whole family gathers together to partake of the same meal. It's the time when dietary restrictions, allergies, preferences, and diets tend to clash with each other, and it can be extremely difficult to cater to all the different tastes and requirements and create a meal that everyone enjoys.

Fortunately, many of these keto recipes are just as tasty as their normal counterparts, and everyone should be able to eat them – adults and children alike. You don't have to cheat on your diet to create a satisfying meal for everyone to enjoy together, and you don't have to cook two separate dinners at the end of a long day.

It's really important to make sure that your dinner is satisfying, because the hours between dinner and bed are the ones where many people choose to start snacking, and that's when it gets harder to stick to your commitments and keep eating healthily. You might also struggle at dinner if you have already used up a lot of your carb allowance during the day, and therefore don't have much left to play with for the evening meal.

Don't despair, because we have some great recipes for you to try!

Keto Macaroni Cheese

Macaroni cheese is a classic comfort food, and it's delightfully popular with kids as well as adults. You can't get much better than this meal, but if you're following a keto diet, pasta is out – and so a classic dish is seemingly off the menu. However, with this recipe, you can carry on enjoying macaroni cheese without the carbs or heavy bloating that usually follows.

Serves: 8

You will need:

- 2 tablespoons of olive oil

- 230 ml / 1 cup of double (heavy) cream

- 510 g / 4 cups of grated cheddar cheese

- 1 tablespoon of hot sauce (omit if you don't like spice)

- 170 g / 6 oz. of cream cheese

- 2 heads of cauliflower

- 450 g / 2 cups of mozzarella

- A little butter for the baking dish

- 30 g / ¼ of a cup of Parmesan (or vegetarian hard Italian cheese) to top with, or extra mozzarella if you prefer

- 110 g / 4 oz. crushed walnuts to top with (or another kind of nut if you prefer)

Method:

1. Preheat your oven to 190 degrees C / 375 degrees F, and grease a large baking dish generously with butter.

2. Cut your cauliflower heads into florets and toss them with the olive oil (plus some salt if you choose).

3. Spread your cauliflower out on a baking sheet (or on several baking sheets) and then roast it for 40 minutes, until it has turned lightly golden.

4. While the cauliflower is roasting, put a pot on a medium heat, and then add the cream. When it begins to simmer, turn down the heat and stir in both your mozzarella and the cheddar (but not the Parmesan/mozzarella intended for topping). Mix and heat until the cheese is fully melted.

5. Add your hot sauce if you are going to use it, and then take the pan off the heat and season if necessary.

6. Stir the roasted cauliflower into the sauce, and then tip it into your prepared baking dish.

7. Mix your Parmesan, crushed walnuts, and oil in a bowl, and then spread the mixture on top of your dish.

8. Place the dish in the hot oven and bake until the top turns golden. This should take about 15 minutes, and then you can turn the oven up to broil for 2 minutes if you like, or serve without crisping the top.

Approximate Nutritional Information For One Serving:

Calories: 610

Fat: 54.8 g

Saturated Fat: 28 g

Cholesterol: 139 mg

Sodium: 629 mg

Total Carbohydrates: 8.1 g

Dietary Fibre: 2.6 g

Total Sugars: 2.4 g

Protein: 25.2 g

Goan Mussels

If you want a rather fancy dinner idea, you can show off to your guests just how great keto can really be with this amazing mussel dish. It's extremely easy and should only take about half an hour to make, but it tastes great, and you can add other seafood options to it if you like. It's worth noting that this isn't the lowest carb dish out there, so it's worth saving on your other meals and making this a treat, rather than an everyday option.

Serves: 4

You will need:

- 400 ml / 1 ½ cups of coconut milk

- 1 large onion

- 1 teaspoon of ground coriander

- 1 teaspoon of ground cumin

- ½ a teaspoon of ground turmeric

- 5 cloves of garlic

- 3 green chillies

- 1 kg / 2.2 lb. of fresh mussels

- 1 inch thumb of ginger

- 1 tablespoon of sunflower oil for frying in

- Lime wedges for serving

- Parsley for serving

Method:

1. Take the beards off the mussels and then wash them thoroughly in a bowl of cold water. Change the water and keep rinsing the mussels in it until it is clear. Tap any mussels that are open on the side and give them a few minutes. If they do not close up, you should throw them away, along with any that have broken shells. These mussels are dead and may be unsafe to eat.

2. Slice the onion and the chillies, grate the ginger, and mince the garlic.

3. Fry the onion in a pan until it is golden, and then tip in the turmeric, cumin, and coriander, followed by the garlic, ginger, and chillies. Add salt and pepper, and cook for a couple of minutes.

4. Pour in the coconut milk and bring the mixture to a boil, and then simmer it lightly for a few minutes to combine the flavours.

5. Add the muscles to the pan and then put the lid on and turn up the heat to bring the whole thing to a high boil. Boil for about 4 minutes, until all the mussels are open.

6. Serve into bowls and slice a lime to be squeezed over the meal.

Approximate Nutritional Information For One Serving:

Calories: 521

Fat: 33.7 g

Saturated Fat: 22.9 g

Cholesterol: 70 mg

Sodium: 743 mg

Total Carbohydrates: 24.1 g

Dietary Fibre: 4.2 g

Total Sugars: 6 g

Protein: 33.6 g

Herby Balsamic Chicken

Chicken is a fantastic meal to make in the evening, because it's a meat that almost everyone enjoys, and in terms of the planet, it's a little bit better than some of the other meats (e.g. beef). All around, it's a great ingredient, because it takes on flavours very well, and it's quick and relatively easy to cook.

Serves: 6

You will need:

- 6 chicken thighs (preferably boneless and skinless)
- 120 ml / 1/2 cup of balsamic vinegar
- 3 teaspoons of lemon zest
- 2 cloves of garlic
- 1 tablespoon of fresh basil
- 1 tablespoon of fresh chives
- 3 tablespoons of olive oil
- Pinch of salt
- Pinch of pepper

Method:

1. Mince the garlic, grate the lemon zest, and finely chop the chives and basil.

2. Get a large bowl and add all of the ingredients except for the chicken. Whisk them together to combine them.

3. Toss the chicken into the vinegar mixture and coat it, and then allow it to sit for 10 minutes in the fridge.

4. Remove the chicken and place it in a skillet and fry it for several minutes. Flip it and fry it for another 6 minutes or so, and then insert a meat thermometer and check that the internal temperature reads at least 80 degrees C / 170 degrees F. When it does, take the chicken out and place it on a plate, and then drizzle the rest of the vinegar mixture across it to serve. You can add some green beans, some broccoli, or some spinach to bulk the meal out and add iron and vitamins if you choose to, or just eat it like this.

Approximate Nutritional Information For One Serving:

Calories: 180

Fat: 12.4 g

Saturated Fat: 2.5 g

Cholesterol: 53 mg

Sodium: 78 mg

Total Carbohydrates: 1.4 g

Dietary Fibre: 0.1 g

Total Sugars: 0.2 g

Protein: 14.8 g

Courgette / Zucchini Pizza

A lot of people find that the hardest thing to give up when they swap to a keto diet is bread — and all the bread-based foods that we enjoy day to day. Pizza is such a classic dinner recipe that you are bound to find yourself tempted by it at times, and unfortunately, it is decidedly too carb-heavy to fit into a keto diet with ease.

However, if your children are pleading for pizza or you just want an easy date-night food, you can still enjoy pizza by making the "bread" your way — and the great news is, this is still easy to freeze and heat up, just like regular pizza. You can choose any toppings that you fancy, as long as they are low in carbs.

Serves: 6

You will need:

- 1 tablespoon of olive oil

- 35 g / $\frac{1}{4}$ cup of flour

- 2 large eggs

- 1 or 1 $\frac{1}{2}$ courgettes / zucchinis

- 45 g / $\frac{1}{2}$ cup of Parmesan (or vegetarian hard Italian cheese)

- 45 g / $\frac{1}{2}$ cup of mozzarella

- 1 tablespoon of fresh basil

- 1 teaspoon of fresh thyme

- 1 sweet red pepper (for the topping)

- 90 g / 1 cup of mozzarella (for the topping)

- 65 g / $\frac{1}{2}$ cup of turkey pepperoni

Method:

1. Preheat your oven to 230 degrees C / 450 degrees F.

2. Shred the courgette / zucchini and squeeze it in a clean towel to remove some of the moisture.

3. Mince the basil and thyme, and slice the sweet red pepper. Lightly beat the eggs.

4. Get a large bowl and mix together the eggs, courgette / zucchini, mozzarella, Parmesan, flour, olive oil, basil, and thyme.

5. Generously grease a 12 inch pizza pan and then spread the mixture out to about an inch from the edges.

6. Place in the oven and bake until the colour turns lightly golden (around 15 minutes). Lower the oven temperature to 200 degrees C / 400 degrees F and take the pizza out of the oven.

7. Add the toppings and sprinkle the cheese on top, and then bake for another 10 minutes or so, until the cheese has all melted.

Approximate Nutritional Information For One Serving:

Calories: 145

Fat: 8.4 g

Saturated Fat: 3.2 g

Cholesterol: 85 mg

Sodium: 366 mg

Total Carbohydrates: 7.8 g

Dietary Fibre: 0.9 g

Total Sugars: 1.7 g

Protein: 10.8 g

Asparagus And Mushroom Frittata

Eggs make a super quick and easy meal, and this frittata is one that kids will love. It's also got plenty of vegetables in it, and if you're rushing to get after school meals on the table, this is one you should definitely learn. You can adapt it to include other vegetables, but mushrooms and asparagus both fit in nicely with the keto diet. It should be ready to eat in about half an hour, and requires very little hands-on prep.

Serves: 8

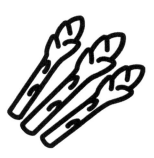

You will need:

- ♦ 9 eggs

- ♦ 2 tablespoons of lemon juice

- ♦ A pinch of salt

- ♦ A pinch of pepper

- ♦ 1 tablespoon of olive oil

- ♦ 65 g / ½ cup of ricotta cheese

- ♦ 2 onions

- ♦ 1 red pepper

- ♦ 30 g of mushrooms

- ♦ 230 g / 8 oz. of asparagus spears

Method:

1.   Slice the red pepper thinly, and then slice the mushrooms and the onions.

2.   Preheat the oven to 175 degrees C / 350 degrees F.

3.   Take a large bowl and whisk together eggs, lemon juice, and ricotta cheese, plus seasoning. You can add other spices here if you want to make the flavours more unusual. Paprika or turmeric make nice additions.

4.   Take a 10 inch, ovenproof skillet, and heat the oil in it.

5.   Add the asparagus, sliced onions, sliced red pepper, and sliced mushrooms and stir them together. Cook them for up to eight minutes, until the pepper and the onion have softened.

6.   Take the pan off the heat and remove the asparagus spears. Cut the spears into short lengths and tip them back into the skillet.

7.   Stir in the egg mixture from the bowl and put the skillet into the oven. Bake it for around 25 minutes and then place it on top of the stove to rest for about 5 minutes. Cut the frittata into portions and serve hot.

Approximate Nutritional Information For One Serving:

Calories: 123

Fat: 7.9 g

Saturated Fat: 2.5 g

Cholesterol: 188 mg

Sodium: 99 mg

Total Carbohydrates: 5.7 g

Dietary Fibre: 1.5 g

Total Sugars: 3 g

Protein: 8.4 g

Healthy Keto Snack Recipes

Sometimes, you just need a snack, and snacking when you're on a diet can be tricky. Snack food has a lot of roles to fulfil. It has to be easy to make, easy to eat, and create minimal mess in the kitchen. It mustn't take hours to create. It has to taste good. It has to satisfy a craving. It's no wonder that most people fall down when it comes to snacks, but you can have snacks that taste great and are still keto.

We're going to run through some of the top options. Avocado might be one of the most popular keto snacks, but there are plenty of other foods that you can choose from if you're not a fan of avocado or you're trying to choose foods that are planet-friendly at the same time as good for you.

Boiled Eggs With Olives And Basil

If you're keen on boiled eggs but a little bored of them, you can try spicing them up with this fantastic recipe. It adds a great twist to the ordinary recipe and makes them a fun, unusual-looking food.

Serves: 12

You will need:

- ♦ 6 large eggs

- ♦ 12 pitted Kalamata olives (or green olives if you prefer)

- ♦ 2 tablespoons of rapeseed oil

- ♦ 1 teaspoon of cider or balsamic vinegar

- ♦ 20 g / 1 packed cup of fresh basil

Method:

1.   Place your eggs in a pan full of cold water and then put the pan on a medium high heat and wait for it to come to a boil. Allow the eggs 8 minutes to cook from the moment when the water starts boiling.

2.   Plunge the eggs into cold water. Refresh the water once or twice, and allow the eggs to cool.

3.   Break the shells and peel the eggs. Cut the eggs in half, and then scoop the yolks out and tip them into a bowl.

4.   Add the vinegar and the oil, and then mince the basil and stir it in. Mash everything together so that the yolks are well combined with the rest of the mixture.

5.   Slice the olives in half and toss them into the bowl, and then scoop the yolk mixture back into the egg whites and serve. If there are any egg halves left over, chill them in the fridge. You should get 12 egg halves from this recipe.

Approximate Nutritional Information For One Serving:

Calories: 64

Fat: 5.3 g

Saturated Fat: 1 g

Cholesterol: 93 mg

Sodium: 73 mg

Total Carbohydrates: 0.5 g

Dietary Fibre: 0.2 g

Total Sugars: 0.2 g

Protein: 3.2 g

Keto Coconut Shortbread

If you've got a craving for something sweet, you might struggle on the keto diet, because sugar can be an issue. That means that many commercially bought biscuits/cookies are out, and so is a lot of chocolate and other snacks. Fortunately, these delicious shortbread cookies are a perfect way to enjoy a sweet treat with a cup of tea or coffee, and the perfect follow-up to any meal.

Serves: 16

You will need:

♦ 30 g / 1/3 of a cup of shredded coconut

♦ 1 teaspoon of coconut extract

♦ 60 g / ½ cup of SPLENDA Sugar Blend for Baking

♦ 12 g / 2 cups of almond flour

♦ 6 tablespoons of butter

Method:

1. Melt the butter in a pan or in the microwave.

2. Mix together the butter, coconut extract, almond flour, and sweetener in a large bowl and stir with a fork until fully combined.

3. Wash your hands and knead the dough lightly, and then form it into an 8 inch log.

4. Wrap the log in cling film / plastic wrap and squeeze it tightly to squash the ingredients together firmly. This will help to ensure that everything combines and sticks together properly.

5. Unroll the wrap and place the log on the counter. Sprinkle the shredded coconut on the log and roll it gently until it is coated with coconut.

6. Rewrap it in plastic and twist the ends up tightly.

7. Place it in the fridge for at least half an hour for the butter to harden. When it has, take it back out and place it on the counter. Get a sharp knife and cut the dough into discs that are a little under an inch thick.

8. Place the discs on a greased baking sheet and preheat your oven to 175 degrees C / 350 degrees F. Bake for up to 15 minutes until it turns golden.

9. Take the shortbread out and let it cool completely before you touch it. Because butter is the only binding ingredient in this recipe, you need to make sure the shortbread is thoroughly cold before you move it.

10. Store in the fridge to keep the butter fresh, or keep in the freezer for up to 6 months.

Approximate Nutritional Information For One Serving:

Calories: 84

Fat: 5.1 g

Saturated Fat: 3.3 g

Cholesterol: 11 mg

Sodium: 31 mg

Total Carbohydrates: 7.9 g

Dietary Fibre: 0.2 g

Total Sugars: 7.7 g

Protein: 0.2 g

Keto Chocolate Brownies

Not everyone counts a brownie as a snack, but when you're on a diet, it's important to have a few "treat foods" you can turn to when you're struggling. Doing so actually makes you more likely to stick to the diet, because you won't be constantly denying yourself – which gives you more staying power. These keto chocolate brownies are therefore a perfect solution that lets you enjoy a bit of chocolatey goodness without ruining the diet.

Serves: 16

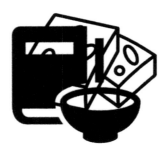

You will need:

- 115 ml / ¹⁄₂ a cup of coconut oil

- 170 g / ³⁄₄ of a cup of sweetener (nutritional information calculated for SPLENDA Sugar Blend for Baking)

- 2 teaspoons of vanilla extract

- 2 eggs

- 170 g / 1 cup of sugar free chocolate

- 2 tablespoons of cocoa powder

- 75 g / 2/3 of a cup of almond flour (not almond meal)

- 85 g / ¹⁄₂ cup of sugar free chocolate chips

Method:

1. Preheat your oven to 180 degrees C / 350 degrees F.

2. Roughly chop up your chocolate so that it is nicely chunked. If you like, you can use extra chocolate instead of chocolate chips.

3. Melt the coconut butter in a small bowl in the microwave in 20 second increments. Add the chocolate to the bowl and stir it in, and then microwave for another 30 seconds. Whisk it to combine, and give it another 10 seconds if the chocolate hasn't fully melted yet.

4. In a different bowl, mix together the cocoa powder and the almond flour.

5. Add the sweetener and the eggs to the melted chocolate and whisk thoroughly, and then tip this mixture into the cocoa and flour bowl. Mix until you have a thick batter, with no lumps.

6. Fold in your chocolate chips, and then tip the mixture into a greased and floured baking tin and transfer it to the oven to bake for 30 minutes.

7. Take the tin out of the oven and allow it to cool before tipping the brownies out and cutting them up. They can be enjoyed cold or gently warmed in the microwave, and should keep for several days in the fridge.

Approximate Nutritional Information For One Serving:

Calories: 171

Fat: 11.4 g

Saturated Fat: 8.1 g

Cholesterol: 23 mg

Sodium: 13 mg

Total Carbohydrates: 18.1 g

Dietary Fibre: 1.1 g

Total Sugars: 10.8 g

Protein: 1.4 g

Crispy Keto Kale Crisps / Chips

Crisps / chips are a tough snack to give up and you will probably find that you miss them at first. There isn't much that will satisfyingly replace them, and sometimes, you just want something salty and crunchy to munch on. If you're struggling with this, it's well worth trying these kale crisps / chips. They aren't the same, but they are a whole lot better for you, and absolutely delicious! You do need an air fryer to make this recipe to perfection, although you can grill kale for a somewhat similar effect if you don't have one.

You should note that kale chips are higher in carbs than most of the other snacks, so keep this one to a minimum and only turn to it for a special treat. It still contains far fewer carbs than a packet of crisps / chips!

Serves: 1

You will need:

♦ ½ tablespoon of olive oil

♦ 200 g / 7 oz. of kale

♦ Pinch of salt

♦ Pinch of pepper

♦ Any other seasoning you wish to add

Method:

1. Wash your kale and chop it into large pieces. Pat it dry on a clean towel and then spread it on a tray. Toss it with the olive oil and season with salt, pepper, and any other flavouring that appeals.

2. Place it in the air fryer basket and cook it for 3 minutes at 200 degrees C / 400 degrees F. Shake the basket and cook for another 2 minutes.

3. Serve the kale and eat it hot, or allow it to cool down to room temperature before enjoying. It will not keep very well, so make small portions as you want them, rather than trying to store the kale.

Approximate Nutritional Information For One Serving:

Calories: 282

Fat: 7 g

Saturated Fat: 1 g

Cholesterol: 0 mg

Sodium: 350 mg

Total Carbohydrates: 21 g

Dietary Fibre: 3 g

Total Sugars: 0 g

Protein: 6 g

Broccoli Tots

A cute snack, broccoli tots look very tempting and they use a super healthy veggie to make delicious little bites of goodness. These can be eaten as a snack or served as a side dish with meals, and they are also vegan and gluten free, making them ideal for anyone. You can add a sprinkling of cheese if you prefer, but remember that they won't be vegan then.

These tots can be eaten hot or cold, and they will also freeze well, making them a great snack to have on hand, especially if you frequently find yourself raiding the kitchen cupboards.

Serves: 4

You will need:

- ♦ 1 clove of garlic
- ♦ ½ cup of almond flour
- ♦ ¼ cup of ground flaxseed
- ♦ 1 teaspoon of salt
- ♦ 450 g / 1 lb. of broccoli

Method:

1. Start by dicing your broccoli florets and stems into small pieces and placing them above a pan of water to steam. If you don't have a steamer, simply put a small amount of water at the bottom of the pan and add the broccoli directly to it. Most of the broccoli will steam, although some will be in contact with the water.

2. Check that the broccoli is tender (this should take approximately 5 minutes, depending on the size of your pieces) and then strain it and put it in your food processor. Pulse it until it is small and rice-like. You can also chop it, but it will not end up as fine and your tots may not stick together as well.

3. Mix together the flaxseed and ground almond in a bowl, and then add the broccoli. Mince the garlic and add this, along with the salt.

4. Stir everything together and allow it to sit for a few minutes. Next, get a baking tray and form the mixture into around 18 tots on the tray. You are aiming for a fat sausage shape, and you should be able to create this simply by using your hands. Make sure you squeeze the mixture together so it doesn't crumble in the oven.

5. Bake at 190 degrees C / 375 degrees F for 15 minutes, and then take the tots out and turn them all over. Bake for another 5 minutes. Both sides should turn golden.

Approximate Nutritional Information For One Serving:

Calories: 107

Fat: 5.5 g

Saturated Fat: 0.4 g

Cholesterol: 0 mg

Sodium: 624 mg

Total Carbohydrates: 11.8 g

Dietary Fibre: 6 g

Total Sugars: 2.1 g

Protein: 5.9 g

Asparagus And Bacon Bites

If you fancy something salty, tasty, and simple, you will love these asparagus bacon bites, which are ultra easy to make and can be whipped up in just half an hour. Again, they make a great snack or a great side dish, and they look fancy too. If you aren't sure about asparagus, try switching it for another vegetable, but you should find the combination between the tender asparagus and the crispy bacon delightful.

Serves: 6

You will need:

- 9 spears of asparagus
- 140 g / 5 oz. of cream cheese
- Pinch of salt
- Pinch of pepper
- 2 cloves of garlic
- 6 slices of bacon

Method:

1. Set your cream cheese on the counter to soften, and chop your bacon strips into thirds.

2. Blanch your asparagus in boiling water so that it is cooked and tender. Drain and set it aside for later use.

3. Preheat your oven to 200 degrees C / 400 degrees F, and grease a baking sheet ready to use.

4. Place a large skillet over a medium heat and then toss in the bacon. Cook it until it is soft – you don't want it to turn too crispy, or you won't be able to wrap it. It does need to be fully cooked, however, so watch it closely. When the bacon is done, place the pieces on a paper towel to drain.

5. Mince your garlic cloves and mix them with the cream cheese, and then season.

6. Once your bacon is cool, spread a little cream cheese on each piece, and then put an asparagus spear on top. Roll the bacon up to completely encircle the cream cheese and asparagus.

7. Do this for each roll, and then place them in the oven and bake them for around 5 minutes, until the bacon has turned crispy.

8. Serve hot and enjoy.

Approximate Nutritional Information For One Serving:

Calories: 191

Fat: 16.1 g

Saturated Fat: 7.7 g

Cholesterol: 47 mg

Sodium: 536 mg

Total Carbohydrates: 2.2 g

Dietary Fibre: 0.5 g

Total Sugars: 0.5 g

Protein: 9.4 g

Meal Prep Tips

One of the keys to following a diet successfully is to make your life as easy as you can, and the best way to make keto easy is to learn some great tricks for preparing meals fast. These can be applied to other situations than the keto diet, but they are ideal for speeding up your kitchen work and maximising the ease with which you can prepare meals.

Use Frozen Foods When You Need To

A lot of people feel that they have to use only fresh, organic, just-picked vegetables when they start a healthy eating diet, and while it's true that fresh vegetables are a great thing to be eating, it's also okay to depend upon frozen ones when necessary.

Sometimes, life is just too busy to be slicing and peeling and preparing everything, and having a bag of your favourite vegetables in the freezer is a great way to deal with this issue. Frozen foods are still highly nutritious, and they are so much easier to cook – you will probably find that your diet actually gets healthier as a result of choosing them, because you will be eating more vegetables overall.

However, you do need to make sure you are choosing your frozen vegetables with care so you aren't getting additives that you don't want or need. Look out for adding salt and sugar, and avoid these frozen foods, or you'll find your carb intake is shooting up again.

Create Portions In Advance

If you have to weigh out your snacks like nuts every single time you want to eat them, it takes a lot longer to grab a quick snack. Calculating carbs is one of the most annoying and time-consuming parts of following the keto diet, but it's important to do, because if you just guess, you'll end up with your numbers totally skewed and your diet failing. You need to know how much of something you are eating.

A great solution to this is to make yourself portions in advance. Get some small bags or airtight plastic tubs and calculate once – and then make yourself a handful of snack pots that are ready to go. If you know that 50 grams of almonds contains 10.7 grams of carbs, you can make your snack pots based on this knowledge, and simply weigh out ingredients.

Being able to just grab a tub from the cupboard and knowing exactly what your carb intake will be makes it so much easier to stick to keto when you're rushing around. You can even write the quantities on the tubs if you're in need of reminders. Keep using the same tubs for the same quantities of food and you'll make this sort of snacking a total breeze.

Freeze Meals

When you've found the perfect meal, it's a great idea to make extra and then freeze the additional portions. This saves you time in the future, and it doesn't take much longer to create a couple of extra portions for yourself. Write the nutritional information on the container so it's easy to balance the meal with whatever else you're eating that day.

You can make yourself very easy lunches by simply freezing some of yesterday's dinner in a container, or have dinner ready for several nights in a row with this method. You'll soon find that you're breezing through the week with minimal cooking because this organisation technique saves you so much time. It also saves on cleaning up! Simply grab a meal from the freezer the night before, let it defrost overnight, and enjoy it the following day.

Of course, not every kind of food freezes well, so it's worth experimenting before you batch cook any recipe. A lot of foods that contain cream or cream cheese don't work brilliantly in the freezer, as the texture tends to change. Foods with a lot of water in, such as tomatoes and cucumbers, also don't taste great after being frozen. However, this is a great hack for most foods and can save you significant amounts of time.

Prepare Vegetables In Advance

You can buy ready-sliced vegetables, but these tend to be expensive, so it's better to prep them yourself if you can. Putting a few hours into washing, cutting, and storing your vegetables in advance can make things much easier when you come to actually cooking – because you can just throw everything in a pan.

This is good if you're working during the week, but you have some free time over the weekend. You can reduce the amount of preparation that needs to be done after work without reducing the number of fresh vegetables that you eat. When the vegetables are already prepared, it's much easier to find the motivation to put together something really healthy.

Of course, not all vegetables keep well if you cut them in advance, so you may only want to prepare enough for a couple of days. Things like peppers, onions, mushrooms, garlic, and courgette / zucchini should be fine cut up in advance, but they will start to turn soft more quickly. Broccoli, cauliflower, and Brussels sprouts should keep better. Make sure you store all sliced vegetables in airtight containers once they have been cut, to minimise the airflow and keep them as fresh as possible.

Learn To Make Great Dressings

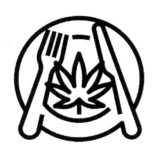

Many commercially available salad dressings are not keto friendly, which can mean that you end up eating boring, dry salads – but you don't have to. It's very easy to make your own dressings at home from a whole range of ingredients, and if you do this, you can start adding them to any meal that you fancy; a good dressing doesn't have to be exclusively reserved for lettuce. Mix some lemon juice, olive oil, salt, and a bit of pepper together, and you've got an instant salad dressing to enjoy.

Create Meal Plans

Often, half of the battle lies in deciding what to eat, so making a meal plan can be a lifesaver. It's also important in terms of calculating your carbs and knowing what to eat. You don't want to choose three carb heavy meals in one day, so make sure you're creating your plan based on the nutritional information.

Remember to factor in snacks and desserts, as well as drinks. This will help to ensure that you stay on track without having to think about it, and makes choosing what to eat a breeze. Some people don't like to stick to a rigid meal plan, in which case having a few options could help. For example, your meal plan might say that you will have mushroom soup or balsamic chicken for dinner.

Allowing yourself some flexibility and choice will help you to stay on track and make the diet more enjoyable. After all, you don't want to turn food into a complete chore, so try to give yourself a little variation and the ability to pick an alternative if you just don't fancy what's on the menu for the day.

Keep Some Pantry Staples In

You can't follow a keto diet if you don't have the basics in. Even if you are a pro at meal prep and you have a meal plan for every day of the week, it's still a good idea to have some backup ingredients that are ideal for whipping up a keto meal with, and you should always make sure your pantry is well stocked with these ingredients.

You should try to have store cupboard ingredients like:

- Mixed nuts
- Mixed seeds
- Cocoa powder
- Vanilla extract
- Vinegar
- Coconut oil
- Coconut flour
- Almond flour
- Baking powder
- Garlic

Keto sweeteners (preferably a variety)

Herbs and spices that you enjoy, such as cinnamon, thyme, red pepper flakes, parsley, etc. You don't want your food to be bland, so have a whole range of herbs and spices ready and try different ones with different meals.

Fridge ingredients should include:
- ❧ Butter
- ❧ Cheeses
- ❧ Eggs
- ❧ Plain yoghurt
- ❧ Coconut milk (full fat)

Having these things to hand will make it much easier to create meals from scratch if you need to suddenly change your dinner plans, so make sure there are always plenty of things in your pantry to choose from.

Conclusion

Following a keto diet can be challenging, but it will be worth it to improve your health and spend every day both feeling and looking better. If you're interested in making a difference to your diet, it's well worth giving it a try, and incorporating these recipes into your kitchen repertoire. Remember to add up totals and ensure that you account for any substitutions you make to keep the nutritional information as accurate as possible.

Use the meal prep tips to simplify your life and make cooking a breeze, and remember that what counts with this sort of diet is the long-term commitment that you make when you start. It's fine to have days in which you don't do as well as you'd hoped and it's fine to have little wobbles. If you keep going, you'll find that it makes the world of difference to how you eat.

Remember that it can take several days to reach a state of ketosis if you've been eating normal foods for a while, so you need to be patient with this diet in order to see results. You won't instantly start burning fat instead of sugar just because you have started eating more healthily; it will take a bit of time for your system to work up to this.

The more closely you can stick to the keto diet, the more quickly you'll see results, and the better you will feel about it all. Make the most of the wonderful array of recipes available to turn your keto diet into something that you can enjoy and feel proud of.

Disclaimer

This book contains opinions and ideas of the author and is meant to teach the reader informative and helpful knowledge while due care should be taken by the user in the application of the information provided. The instructions and strategies are possibly not right for every reader and there is no guarantee that they work for everyone. Using this book and implementing the information/recipes therein contained is explicitly your own responsibility and risk. This work with all its contents, does not guarantee correctness, completion, quality or correctness of the provided information. Misinformation or misprints cannot be completely eliminated.

Printed in Great Britain
by Amazon

80292866R00066